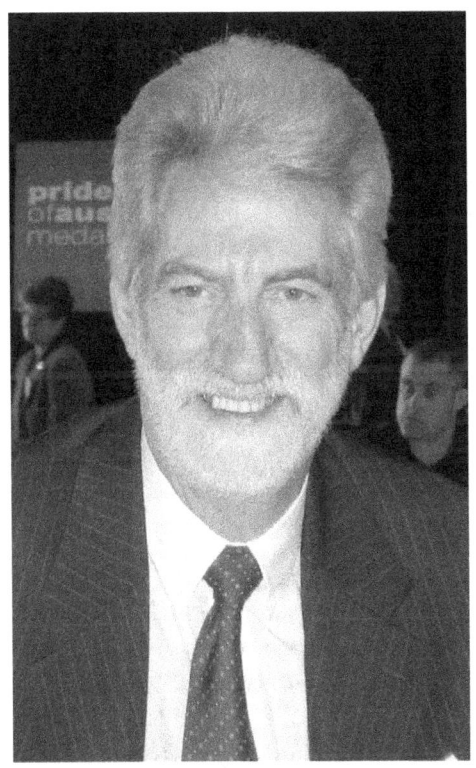

John Coleman, ND , Naturopath

Table of Contents

John Coleman, ND , Naturopath.. 1

It is my pleasure to interview John Coleman, a naturopath doctor from Melbourne, Australia, who was diagnosed with Parkinson's in 1995 but has no symptoms today. Please tell us about your history with Parkinson's John. 5

So you were in pretty bad shape in 1995 in terms of symptoms? 6

How did you come to the realization you could get better when all indications were that you would get worse? 7

There is so much information out there about what is supposed to help – vitamins, supplements, body therapies, etc. etc. How did you go about deciding what to try in terms of therapies, supplements, doctors, etc.? 8

Interview with John Coleman, ND

It sounds like the approach really was to be methodical and sequential so that you would try one approach and see what the effect was and then move on to something else rather than trying a group of therapies all at the same time?... 9

Which therapies/approaches did not work for you? 9

What has helped you get the most relief from your own symptoms? 10

Are you cured?... 10

As a naturopath, do you cure people with Parkinson's?................................... 11

What does your neurologist say about your own remission?........................... 11

Do you personally still do all the things you talk about in your book, Stop Parkin' and Start Livin' (Bowen therapy, Aquas, diet, meditation, supplements, etc.) . 11

Could you say a little more about the Aquas? Many people will not know what you are talking about. 12

What would happen if you stopped doing all these things you talk about in your book? Does a point in time come when you can just stop doing all this stuff?. 13

What do you recommend for pain? 13

What do you recommend for anxiety?... 14

What do you recommend for the inability to sleep? 15

What do you recommend for depression? 16

What do you recommend for constipation?... 17

What do you recommend for tremors?.. 18

When I talk about Parkinson's at Parkinson's support groups I always talk about your recovery. At one of my recent talks a man said to me "He never had

Interview with John Coleman, ND

Parkinson's to begin with. No one recovers from Parkinson's." Is it possible this man is right and you were actually misdiagnosed in 1995?.............................. 19

What is the most important thing you want people to know who have Parkinson's? 22

What was recovery like for you? Once you started on the road to recovery doing all the things that do help relieve symptoms did you get a little bit better every day? Or are there blocks of time - 1 day, 1 week, 1 month, several months - when you actually feel worse?.. 22

What about your patients… what has their experience been like?................... 23

Among your patients with Parkinson's, how many are getting relief from their symptoms? How many have been able to see full relief from their symptoms? 24

Does a person have to make any lifestyle changes to recover?........................ 25

It took you three and a half years to recover. That is a long time to sustain hope. How did you do it? 25

Of the people you see initially, about what proportion is unwilling to make the lifestyle changes that are necessary to recover?... 26

Do you do individual consultations? How would this work for people who do not live in Australia? How do people get in touch with you?.................................. 27

If people want to join your mentoring program is that something that lasts six months, a year, two years. Is it flexible? How does it work exactly?................ 28

Do you have any information regarding the supplement NADH that is supposed to improve cognitive abilities? Does it interfere with Azilect (or Rasagiline)? .. 29

How can I reduce or manage my rigidity, spasms and burning sensations? Please advise me. 32

Interview with John Coleman, ND

How many people have undertaken the same plan and what results have they gotten? 34

When should we start taking medication? 38

Could you discuss the approaches using the Emotional Freedom Technique for my Parkinson's condition and your opinion of the value of the technique? 40

I take Mirapex three times a day; also Carbidopa/levodopa three times a day. Which should be taken first and when? How critical is the timing of taking medication? 42

How do I handle the negativity (Doomsday) when keeping my appointment with the neurologist? 44

In Your 12 Step Recovery Program, are some steps more important than others? 48

Step 1: Understanding How Parkinson's Disease Develops 48

Step 2 - Loving Ourselves 49

Step 5 – Laughter 50

Step 7 – Meditating 50

Step 6 – Diet 51

Does your 12 Step Recovery Program interfere or complement electric Deep Brain Stimulation (DBS)? 51

Given that you worked in a copper mine at age 16 suggests metal poisoning caused your Parkinson's. A chemist says, once rid of the metal, your body recovered. Most don't have such a traceable cause. Your method healed you, yet may not transfer to others? 54

Interview with John Coleman, ND

Over the last few days there have been results of studies suggesting that there can be benefits of early medication rather than delaying medication. Comments? 56

How long did it take you see substantial symptom relief? How long did it take to become symptom free? 58

Could you say a little about your 12 Step Recovery Program? 61

About Parkinsons Recovery 62

Index 62

Reference 68

It is my pleasure to interview John Coleman, a naturopath doctor from Melbourne, Australia, who was diagnosed with Parkinson's in 1995 but has no symptoms today. Please tell us about your history with Parkinson's John.

In retrospect I can tell you that I had a long journey developing symptoms. I actually can recognize some of my symptoms from my mid teens. This was particularly true of my twenties when I started to develop an intermittent tremor and I had a lot of trouble with stiffness in my hip and back and neck. I tended to ignore these symptoms as you do when we are young. I went to

a chiropractor occasionally but, most of the time I just told my body what I wanted it to do. I tended to be a busy, high achiever type person, worked two or three jobs at a time, brought up a family, renovated a house all at the same time, but I had a number of very stressful times in my life and I know that symptoms tended to escalate.

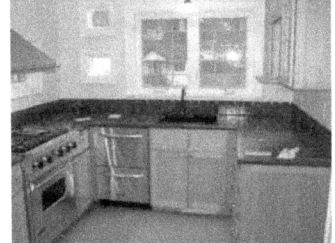

Interview with John Coleman, ND

For instance, my older son's illness and subsequent death in 1983. Separation of my first marriage. I was unemployed for some time. During these periods I knew that my body was rebelling but did not want to take any notice of physical symptoms. I was a cigarette smoker for 43 years. That may make me seem very old, but I actually started when I was 9 years old.

One of the things in my background is a very abusive childhood. I tried to commit suicide when I was 9 and failed, so I started smoking and that helped build a smokescreen.

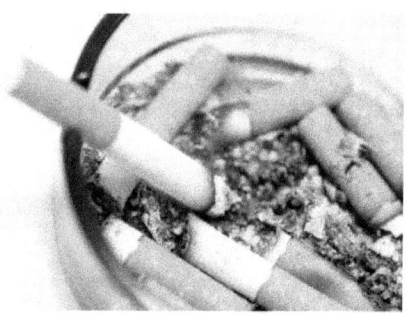

We know that nicotine disguises the onset of Parkinson's. It makes it appear we are actually less symptomatic than we are.

When I stopped smoking in 1995, and my body lost that nicotine support, my symptoms started to escalate more quickly until in the middle of 1995 when I collapsed. It was just impossible for me to ignore my body any longer.

So you were in pretty bad shape in 1995 in terms of symptoms?

John: Yes I was. I was in a state of total meltdown.

I was unable to walk more than 3-5 meters.

I needed support when walking.

I fell often.

I had very, very severe tremor.

I was not sleeping.

I was in a lot of pain.

Interview with John Coleman, ND

My face was frozen.

I was dribbling from my mouth uncontrollably.

I was incontinent and constipated.

It was difficult for me to get up from a chair.

I froze. I would be walking and try and turn a corner and I couldn't. I would just freeze on the spot.

There were a lot of very bad things happening to me which I realize, thinking back, had been coming on a long time but I had ignored them.

> **How did you come to the realization you could get better when all indications were that you would get worse?**

I didn't know. I had no indication that I could get better. What I knew was that I had to make each day better than the last because I couldn't survive the way I was. I set about achieving something every day.

Survival was a good thing each day. Because frankly Robert, I thought I was dying, as did many people around me. I knew it was my responsibility to make a choice to fade away or to make each day better. No one else could do it for me and there was no one else around who was willing to do it for me. I just survived each day and did the best I could.

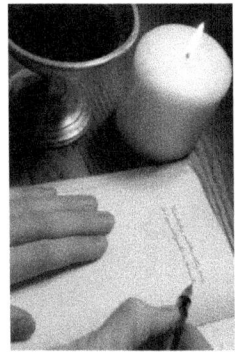 *I kept journals. Over a long period of time I started to see, reading my journals, that I was actually making improvements in my health. That gave me some hope to make each day a bit better than the last.*

7

Interview with John Coleman, ND

> **There is so much information out there about what is supposed to help – vitamins, supplements, body therapies, etc. etc. How did you go about deciding what to try in terms of therapies, supplements, doctors, etc.?**

Trial and error and mainly error. I was becoming aware of how my body responded to various remedies and therapies. I had a history with chiropractors and osteopaths, so I was aware of that sort of response.

So what I did was try one thing at a time. Make one change and observe what happened. Then I changed another thing.

I was also studying naturopathy so that I was aware of the complementary health theory of dealing with degeneration, so I tried things like Vitamin CError! Bookmark not defined., Vitamin E, coenzyme Q10, picnoginal, etc and gave myself a time frame with each one. So I would try it for a period of time and make some observations. If you like I was a research population of one for myself.

I was working for a major hospital at the time here in Melbourne, as an

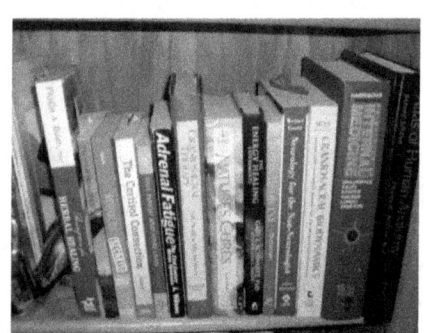 *operating theatre technician, so I had access to the hospital medical library. I did an enormous amount of research there with the cooperation of the hospital staff who were very kind to me. I examined hundreds of abstracts and full studies, trying to find anything that would say to me "this will help."*

I just kept on trying and trying and trying until I found some things that helped me improve my health.

Interview with John Coleman, ND

It sounds like the approach really was to be methodical and sequential so that you would try one approach and see what the effect was and then move on to something else rather than trying a group of therapies all at the same time?

John: Ideally yes. I wasn't always logical and sometimes jumped from one thing to another. One of the things in my favor, though it did not seem so at the time, was that I was pretty much broke. It quickly became apparent that I had to sell my little house that I owned just to pay for therapies. I wasn't earning much money. I just had to try one thing at a time, generally because that was all that I could afford, and that was a good thing.

Which therapies/approaches did not work for you?

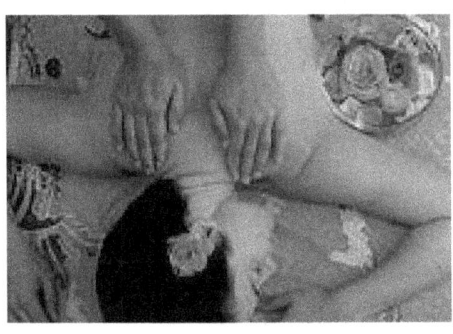

There were a lot. In general, any form of bodywork that was firm or hard - so deep tissue massage, sports massage – those sorts of massages created extra pain. Vigorous therapies like chiropractic and other manipulative therapies also tended to increase my symptoms and create pain.

Excessive intake of nutritional supplements tended to have no effect or make me nauseous or simply be a waste of money. I had to be very careful about homeopathic remedies because the normal approach in selecting potencies and frequencies seemed to aggravate me where a very gentle, a very cautious approached worked.

Many counseling modalities helped. Psychiatry did not. I am sure there are good psychiatrists out there, but I saw four and none of them helped me at all.

Antidepressant therapy did not work. I choose not to take pharmaceuticals, but other forms of herbal, vitamin homeopathic remedies for depression, but I realized I actually was not depressed. I was certainly anxious, but the antidepressant therapies were just no good for me. I needed to be active and proactive in my approach.

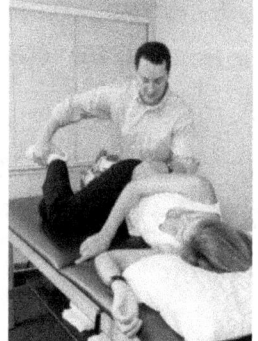

In general, anything that was too hard, too vigorous, too enthusiastic didn't work, and gentle, cautious, loving therapies worked.

What has helped you get the most relief from your own symptoms?

This is very hard to define individually. It is really a whole package. What I did was focus on improving my health in every possible way: physically, emotionally, mentally and spiritually. I intuitively knew this whole package approach was the only way I was going to get out of the hell hole I was in at the time.

I knew it was up to me to change and I had to change virtually everything and make every aspect of my life better. As I did that, the symptoms faded.

I did not focus on symptoms. I looked at what was in my life that needed to be changed, and worked with that. Then the symptoms slowly disappeared.

Are you cured?

No. I do not believe in cure and no I am not cured. But I have recovered my health. That is a very different thing. I have chosen to lead a life that is healthy and loving. The reward for that is that my body displays good health.

Interview with John Coleman, ND

As a naturopath, do you cure people with Parkinson's?

No. I do not cure anybody of anything. Nobody can cure Parkinson's disease, and I certainly can't.

However, I can use my experience and research, and the research from elsewhere around the world, to guide other people diagnosed with Parkinson's into a healthier lifestyle that, if they are dedicated to that process, may enable them to recover their health, and will certainly improve their health and their quality of life.

What does your neurologist say about your own remission?

The professor of neurology who saw me in 1995 and 1996 apologized for his treatment of me some five years after my recovery. Then, after he retired from practice, I approached him to speak at a meeting of the Neuro Recovery Foundation. He called back to congratulate me on my health and on the work I was doing, but chose not to speak and has chosen not to speak publicly about my experience or my recovery.

Do you personally still do all the things you talk about in your book, Stop Parkin' and Start Livin' (Bowen therapy, Aquas, diet, meditation, supplements, etc.)

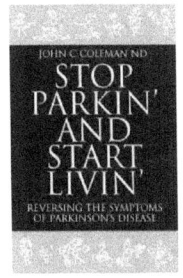

I do most of them. We have to recognize that Stop Parkin' and Start Livin' was written for people who are in the throes of Parkinson's disease. I now have no symptoms yet I still choose to do most of the things.

I meditate daily. I start my day with meditation.

I exercise daily.

Interview with John Coleman, ND

I use affirmations and mirror-talk to assure myself of my power and beauty.

My wife Nichol and I spend a lot of time laughing, and I look for humor in 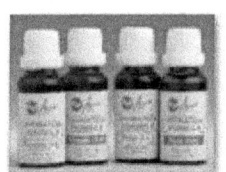 *what I do and in my daily life.*

We eat a very healthy diet outlined in the book; that is no wheat, no dairy, high intake of vegetables, some fish, avocado – those sorts of foods – good protein intake.

I still take the Aquas but only twice a week. I feel that is enough for what I require in my healthy state.

I take some basic nutritional supplements to make up for deficiencies in our food supply.

I choose to live a life that has times for rest and reflection, time for me to spend in the garden, time for me to just sit and be.

So yes, I do most of the things in Stop Parkin' and Start Livin' because I choose to be healthy.

> **Could you say a little more about the Aquas? Many people will not know what you are talking about.**

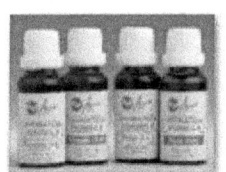
The Aquas, that is the short name for Aqua Hydration Formulas, are homeopathic complex formulas developed in Australia in the 90's. These are remedies that change the way our hypothalamus (a control center in our brain) responds to our environment. This change helps us reduce the production of stress hormones and increase production of neurotransmitters, like dopamine, through the redistribution of fluids around the cell membrane. They are powerful homeopathic remedies that I feel is one of the core therapies for recovery and good health.

Interview with John Coleman, ND

What would happen if you stopped doing all these things you talk about in your book? Does a point in time come when you can just stop doing all this stuff?

Every day we have a choice to make. We can choose to live a life that is healthy or a life that is unhealthy. This is the case whether we're diagnosed with some form of disorder or not. We still have that choice.

I choose to live a life that will enhance my health. If I made a different choice – if I made choices such as I made prior to my collapse – working long silly hours, allowing myself to be stressed out, eating bad food, drinking too much coffee, focusing on negatives – then I would get sick.

I don't know what particular form that particular illness would take – whether I would develop symptoms of Parkinson's again, whether I would develop something like a cancer or Crohn's disease or diabetes – I do not know. But I am certain that I would get sick.

Occasionally I forget about being healthy. I dedicate myself to my clients. I work longer hours than I should and perhaps I don't exercise as much, or I eat on the run. Then my body reacts by saying slow down. I'll get a headache. I'll feel really tired. Maybe I'll feel unwell and that is a reminder to me to make different choices, to spend a little time out. Meditate. Walk. Eat some better food. Drink more water. Then I can feel my health returning.

I have a choice every day, as we all do, to live healthy or live sick. I choose to live well.

What do you recommend for pain?

Depending on the source and type of pain, helpful remedies may be magnesium powders, Bowen Therapy, homeopathic remedies, exercise, laughter, water and

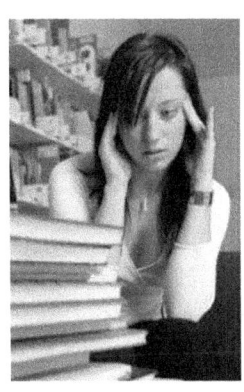

13

© Parkinsons Recovery

sleep. Pain is a very individual symptom. It can occur in many forms and in many areas of our body. We need to understand what the pain is, what type of pain it is, where it is located and what is causing it before getting too enthusiastic about a remedy. For instance, many people come to me and say they have constant headaches. Often all they have to do is increase their water intake from zero to three or four glasses a day and the headache goes away.

There are other sources of pain, other types of pain associated with neurological changes, and that requires working with our total health until the pain goes away as a natural consequence of becoming healthier. It is not a specific answer. It is a very individual challenge.

What do you recommend for anxiety?

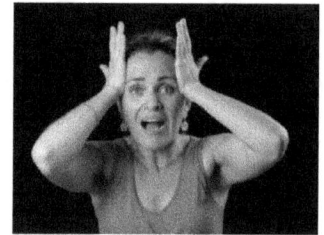

Anxiety usually occurs because there is something for us to be worried about and we are not sure how to deal with it. Some remedies that can help this sort of situation are flower essences, a homeopathic remedy called Trauma/Post Trauma that is made in Australia and available readily, some herbal remedies, and some nutritional supplements can help.

Often we can reduce or eliminate the anxiety through self-help like, for example, meditation or visualization - playing a situation that makes us anxious with a positive outcome. Or, we may require some help from counselors or kinesiologists or some body workers. Anxiety always has a reason and we need to find the reason to deal with it.

Interview with John Coleman, ND

What do you recommend for the inability to sleep?

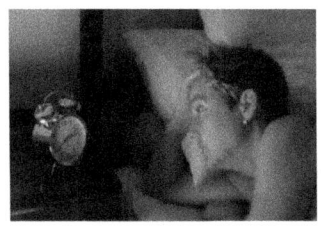

Now this is a difficult challenge for those of us with Parkinson's Disease symptoms. A poor sleep pattern can result from pain, restlessness, a neurotransmitter imbalance between serotonin and melatonin, adrenal stimulation, lack of exercise or lack of fresh air. It seems weird sometimes because we can – in fact we often do – feel really tired to the point of exhaustion. Yet we go to bed and cannot go to sleep or, if we go to sleep we wake frequently.

Some of the things that can help are meditation before bed – say 10 minutes; there are some really good CD's to help that if we need that; some of them can be played softly in the bedroom or some can be listened to through stereo headphones.

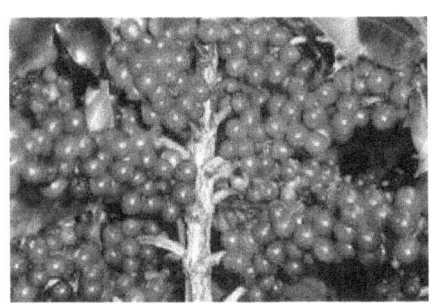

Magnesium powder taken after dinner sometimes helps settle restlessness so that we go to sleep easier. Homeopathic magnesium phosphate or some other homeopathic remedies like coffea or chamomilla can help you sleep. Herbal mixtures like Passionflower, Hops, Jamaica Dogwood can help. One of the important aspects of this is to not become worried or anxious about the lack of sleep because that then sets up a negative feedback pattern. Our sleep pattern becomes even worse.

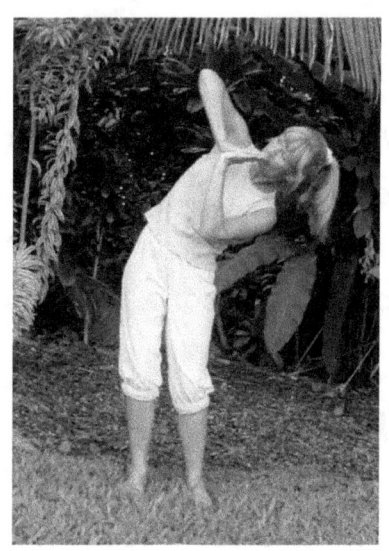

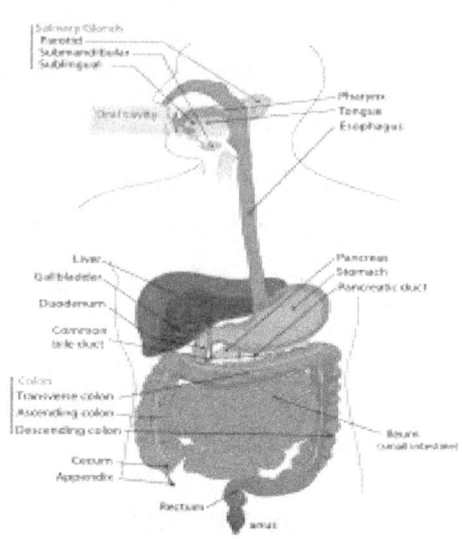

We need to move around during the day as much as we can, particularly if we can get outside, that is good. Keep physically active. We need to get as much fresh air as we can. Make sure we do some stretches before bed to relax our muscles. Often we will sit all evening and then get up and go to bed. Our muscles have gotten quite tight and short so we can't get comfortable. If we do some stretching, some Pilates stretching, or yoga stretching or simple stretching before bed, that will often help our muscles relax better.

It is also really important not to just turn off the television and go to bed. Television stimulates bursts of neurotransmitters in our brain that sets up sort of a chattery situation. If we just switch off the television and go to bed our mind is still chattery. It is important to have 10 minutes or so of quiet time, after we have switched off the television, before we go to bed and go to sleep.

What do you recommend for depression?

Most depression is misdiagnosed in my opinion. I feel that most people with Parkinson's disease are not truly depressed but are anxious about their health and all the negative rubbish

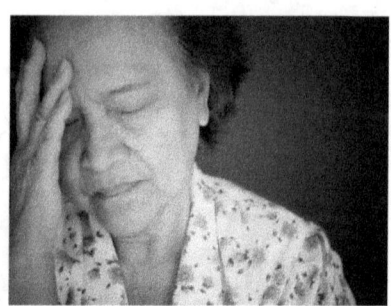

they have been told by the doctors and their relatives and their well-meaning friends.

I have found that this state of anxiety responds well to activity, that is regular exercise, yoga, Pilates, Tai Chi, gardening – just getting out there. Other helpful remedies are flower essences and meditation, especially meditating with affirmations and visualizations.

It's also really important to repair our gastrointestinal tract. A lot of depressive feelings and so-called diagnosed depression result from very poor digestion. If we have poor nutrition, we can't produce the amino acids and the neurotransmitters we need to feel good. Repairing our gastrointestinal tract and eating a really good diet will certainly alleviate depression.

What do you recommend for constipation?

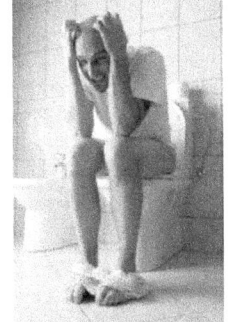

Constipation is very important. This can also have something to do depressive feelings. However in situations like people with Parkinson's, a lot of constipation is created by bowel dehydration. First we need to drink enough water, which is about 1.5 liters or three pints of water daily. Then we can use supplements like Vitamin C and magnesium in powder form, because they will help guide water into the stool and soften it and help us to pass it better. The magnesium encourages peristalsis movement; that is the pulsation of the gut that moves the stool through.

Now if that doesn't work, a naturopath or herbalist could prescribe some nice liquid herbs that will often help. Sometimes that is all that is needed. Sometimes often just drop doses or 3 milliliters of herbal remedies. If necessary, small amounts of fruit laxatives you can get from the health food sections of supermarkets or local health food stores. We have a laxative called _Nulax_ in Australia which is simply compressed fruit. That can help although I wouldn't become reliant on that.

Exercise is very important; exercise like walking, cycling, crawling - all help to move the stool along and get peristalsis working again. There are some specific _Bowen therapy_ moves that can help. I know there are some _yoga_ that are intended to move fecal matter. From experience I know that some of the _Pilates_ and exercises will also help bowel function.

What do you recommend for tremors?

I actually do not worry about tremors. I know a lot of people do. But I believe that tremors are just a superficial symptom indicating our body is uncomfortable. Now I am certain that anyone aware of their body responses notices that when they are calm and peaceful, the tremor reduces 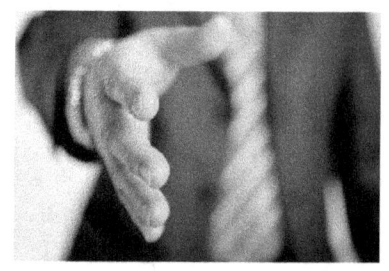 or perhaps goes away entirely. When they are anxious or stressed, the tremor gets worse. This is showing us the fluctuating production of stress hormones from the adrenal glands and the production of dopamine, serotonin and anandamide and so forth, which influence our tremor.

Meditation will certainly help. Laughter will help. Regular exercise will help. All reduce our tendency to tremor. _Bowen therapy_ can help us too. Again improving our general health will reduce our tendency to tremor.

My major advice is don't worry about your tremor. Get well. Then the tremor will disappear.

Interview with John Coleman, ND

> **When I talk about Parkinson's at Parkinson's support groups I always talk about your recovery. At one of my recent talks a man said to me "He never had Parkinson's to begin with. No one recovers from Parkinson's." Is it possible this man is right and you were actually misdiagnosed in 1995?**

To answer that question fully I need to explain what Parkinson's disease is and also how it is diagnosed. Then we can understand it.

Parkinson's is a collection of symptoms first described by James Parkinson 1817, and then expanded by researchers over the following 190 years.

While we tend to focus on well-known symptoms like the tremor, slow movements or the mask-like face, there are many other symptoms that result in a diagnosis of Parkinson's disease. It is interesting that only about 60% of those diagnosed have a tremor.

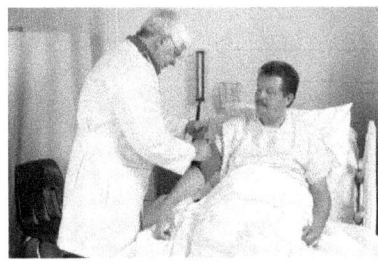

We are diagnosed with Parkinson's disease if we display an accepted group of symptoms that seem to be Parkinson's, the onset of those symptoms is reasonably slow and unilateral, and there is no other explanation for those symptoms.

In 1995 I displayed all the major symptoms of Parkinson's plus many minor symptoms identified as part of this disorder. My symptoms included tremor with pill rolling (that is a very significant hallmark of Parkinson's tremor), I had a masked face, a festinating walk, slow movements, freezing; and the symptoms came on unilaterally prior to spreading to the other side of my body, but they were still more prominent on my right side. They had come on over a long period of time as I explained. All of these, with many other symptoms, pointed to Parkinson's.

Interview with John Coleman, ND

A number of examinations followed that. A physician at my hospital gave me a very thorough workup that included coordination tests, speech tests, hearing, reflexes and so on. He recognized Parkinson's and referred me to a Professor of Neurology. The Professor took five months and a number of visits before he was willing to give me a good examination.

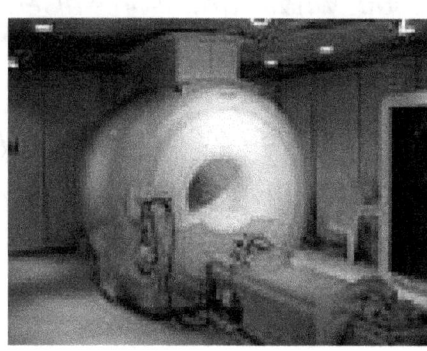

In the meantime I had an MRI scan that showed I had no stroke, no tumor, no MS, no ALS, or any other explanation for the symptoms that we could discern. I was tested for Wilson's disease and in my history there was no contact with any chemicals or drugs that could create all these symptoms of Parkinson's.

During the five months of my visits to the Professor of Neurology, I visited a neurosurgeon who I thought may be able to help me. He gave me a very thorough examination, checked my MRI, checked my history, did all the neuro tests of coordination, etc. and in the end said "you have Parkinson's" unequivocally. He had worked with me in operating theaters for 2 years and he knew me pretty well. We had quite a respect for each other. He understood I was a pretty feet-on-the-ground sort of guy and that this was a real disorder and all of his examinations said Parkinson's.

Later on – five months after my first visit – I went back to the Professor of Neurology who then examined me thoroughly, checked my history again, checked the MRI again, and said "oh, yes. I think it is advanced Parkinson's with early stage multiple system atrophy."

Now that is as good as it gets with diagnosis. There is no specific test or biopsy that can say we have Parkinson's disease. A diagnosis is always the best guess the doctors can make given the circumstances.

Interview with John Coleman, ND

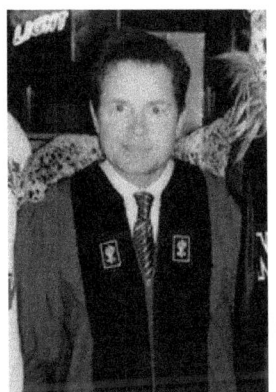

So for instance, there is no hard proof that Michael J. Fox has Parkinson's disease, or Muhammad Ali or anybody at the Parkinson's support groups that you visit. The process for diagnosis for them is the same as it was for me, ending in an educated guess that we have this set of symptoms that we choose to call Parkinson's Disease.

Doctors use two other diagnostic criteria that are actually self-serving. Your gentleman at your support group used one of those criteria. The first is a good response to Levodopa drugs. However, not everyone diagnosed with Parkinson's has a good response to Levodopa drugs and yet they are still diagnosed with Parkinson's Disease. Sometimes – in fact in many cases - doctors will not prescribe Levodopa drugs and yet still diagnose Parkinson's Disease. The interesting thing is that, if we take Parkinson's drugs long enough, we will develop the symptoms of Parkinson's anyway because that is what the drugs do.

The other criteria they use is a failure to get well and continued degeneration. Now that is very self-serving because that means, if somebody gets well, all they need to do is say they must have been misdiagnosed. It was not that many years ago when doctors were saying that about people who recovered from so called incurable cancer. Yet, they continued to recover. Now oncologists understand people can genuinely have what may be thought to be incurable cancer and yet, through their own efforts, become well.

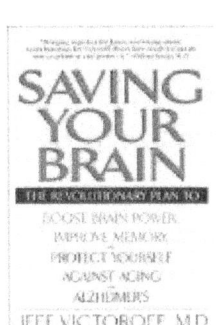

We now know from a huge amount of research, that is not just mine – but research by Jeff Victoroff, Gabor Mate, Norman Doidge, that people can – by understanding the process of Parkinson's - can make changes that will reverse this process.

21

Interview with John Coleman, ND

The short answer is no; I am certain that the diagnosis was correct, and I am certain that I have recovered.

What is the most important thing you want people to know who have Parkinson's?

I want to say to everyone diagnosed with Parkinson's it's your life, your body and your symptoms. Take control and change things. You can choose to live a healthier life. When you do, your body will become healthier.

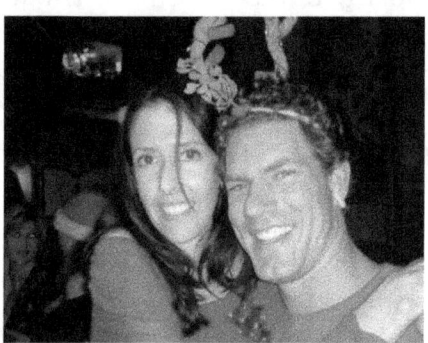

Don't listen to anyone who says you can't. In fact, delete "can't" from your vocabulary. You CAN change if you choose to, and healthy changes will make you healthier.

What was recovery like for you? Once you started on the road to recovery doing all the things that do help relieve symptoms did you get a little bit better every day? Or are there blocks of time - 1 day, 1 week, 1 month, several months - when you actually feel worse?

For me it was a staggering, stumbling time of recovery and discovery, loss, joyfulness, anxiety, despair and sometimes hopelessness. I would start one thing that would seem to help, then I would find it didn't help. Or, I would try something else that would set me back.

I seemed to make slow, fluctuating but OK progress through 1996. Then I had a huge setback. I had back spasms. I was thrown into just incredible despair. I clawed my way out of that and made very fluctuating progress through to the middle of 1997. By that time I was able to speak reasonably coherently and walked reasonably well... didn't fall too often.

Interview with John Coleman, ND

In the middle of 1997 again I had a really huge setback that sent me into black despair. I really contemplated ending it all at that stage. I eventually discovered the [Aquas](#) / [Bowen therapy](#) combination and I found that supported all the other things I was doing like my daily meditation, the counseling that was happening, the self affirmations, my stretching and so on. That gave me real hope.

And remember, I also kept journals right through the time. Intuitively I started keeping a journal within a couple of weeks of my collapse. I think, initially, because I wanted my son to have some sort of record of this part of my life. When I read back on my journals, I could see that, no matter how stumbling and uncertain it seemed, I actually was making some progress toward better health.

What about your patients... what has their experience been like?

I have to say it has been a bit easier for them because I made a lot of the mistakes for them. I was my own guinea pig.

Their health fluctuates a lot because we are very much influenced by what is happening around us in every aspect of our lives. Life is not a straight line or straight path. Any changes in how we live will have ups and downs and uncertainties. They affect our symptom expression.

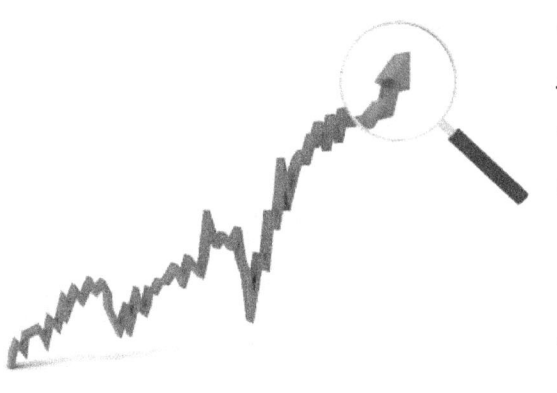

Some of my patients have had times of fantastic progress with letdowns, and struggled back up. Some have had more gentle fluctuations. But, the easier path for them I guess is that they can call me and they have each other. Some patients are setting up networks. They can talk with each other and support each other through

progress toward better health.

> **Among your patients with Parkinson's, how many are getting relief from their symptoms? How many have been able to see full relief from their symptoms?**

The last detailed survey we did was in 2004, mainly because it takes a lot of time and money to do these detailed surveys. That data from 2004 shows that just under 95% of patients were benefiting from the flexible protocol that I advise. This varied from getting slightly better (around 10%) to getting much better (around 80%). Many of those people were able to reduce the western medication or, in a couple of cases, cease medication altogether, and had more robust health.

Only four people other than myself have fully recovered to the extent that they have absolutely no symptoms. That is disappointing. However, we do tend to achieve the health we expect to achieve.

Many people believe that they can get only a bit better so that is what they do. And many people say to me, "If I don't get any worse I will be happy". So what happens is they tend to stay the same. They don't get any worse and they don't get any better because they is what they are expecting, that is what they are aiming for.

I am doing some research now which hopefully will enhance that. We are getting good results. I would like to see better.

Interview with John Coleman, ND

Does a person have to make any lifestyle changes to recover?

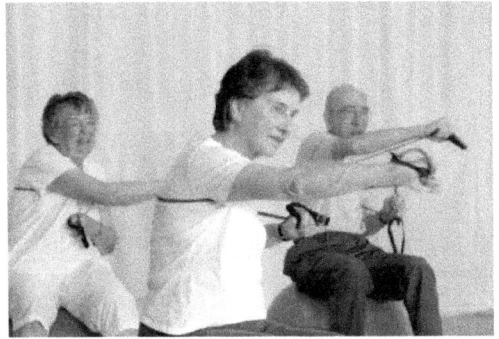

Yes. Unequivocally yes. There is an old saying "if you always do what you have always done, you will always get what you've always got".

Our old lifestyle helped make us sick. We have to change our old lifestyle if we are going to get well. We have to change everything: the way we think; the way we live; the way we relate to the world and the people around us. Yes, we have to change.

It took you three and a half years to recover. That is a long time to sustain hope. How did you do it?

I didn't always have hope. Sometimes I got lost in the misery of my existence and I just wanted to end it.

I had a dream to finish my naturopathic studies before I died. That seems melodramatic but that was really me. I never finished any form of education in my life. I started some courses but through the lack of motivation or the lack of opportunity I had not been able to finish. I desperately wanted to finish this one qualification even if it was the last thing I did.

I kept clawing my way back to functional existence. My journals were very valuable in showing me that over three months or six months or 12 months I was actually showing a trend toward better health. That helped keep me going too.

Another point that was in my favor, although it didn't seem so at the time, was that I lived virtually alone. I actually shared a house with another person who lived up one end of the house. I lived at the other end and we had very little contact. So I was virtually living on my own. I had to do everything for myself.

If I was hungry I had to get the food. If I was dirty I had to wash. If I needed anything I had to get it for myself. That spurred me on to learning how to do it – redeveloping skills and redeveloping strength. Overtime I got to know that I could do something and I kept building on that. I have often said to people my recovery resulted from approximately equal parts of dedication, meditation, hydration and desperation.

Of the people you see initially, about what proportion is unwilling to make the lifestyle changes that are necessary to recover?

I think we have to face the fact that about 80% of the population do not want to take any responsibility for their health. They want a doctor or another practitioner to give them some form of medicine to take the symptoms away, and that is as far as they are willing to go.

Of those who make the effort – and it is a courageous effort to contact me – about 50% drop out pretty quickly because they are unwilling to change a lifetime of bad habits.

They even try to negotiate with me. They say

"Can I have just two coffees a day?"

"Is it OK if I have donuts with morning tea? It is Ok isn't it?"

"I cannot give up my cheese ... anything else but I cannot give up my cheese."

They are prepared to take some drops, some Bowen therapy, exercise a bit, maybe tweak their diet a little bit, but they won't give up their most poisonous habits like coloring their hair, using nail polish, cleaning toilets *with strong bleach, spraying their garden with herbicides or pesticides. They are not prepared to change that.*

Some people face real opposition from their families; siblings, children, partners sometimes are not willing to support the changes required, so make it too hard for their loved one to recover. Sometimes it satisfies some sort of need for a family member.

Sometimes they are just selfish. For instance one of my patients had to stop seeing me because his wife insisted on buying new curtains for the lounge room and he couldn't afford both.

My reward is the small percentage of people who become dedicated to their health and I see them blossom in all aspects of their lives. I have patients who never need to see me again but they keep in contact just to say hi, I am still doing well. That is very rewarding.

> **Do you do individual consultations? How would this work for people who do not live in Australia? How do people get in touch with you?**

Yes. I see people in my clinic in Melbourne. For those in other parts of Australia or other countries there are two options. Firstly, I have a fairly new mentoring program via a web site that I call the 12 Step Recovery Program which offers weekly e-Classes to guide members through all the activities, remedies and therapies that can help them get well.

The other option is to contact me by email or telephone and we do what I call a mail consultation. I provide an extensive questionnaire for completion that I then assess and provide a guidebook with individual advice and prescriptions. It is a bit cumbersome but it has worked pretty well over the last 8 or 9 years before we began our mentoring program.

The easiest way for people to contact me outside of Australia is by my website www.returntostillness.com.au or e-mail me at pdfree@returntostillness.com.au or if they want to telephone it is: +613 9850 9048.

> **If people want to join your <u>mentoring program</u> is that something that lasts six months, a year, two years. Is it flexible? How does it work exactly?**

It is flexible. It is designed to last a 12 month period with weekly lessons, so 52 classes. People can join up and drop out at any point they choose. I am hopeful that, once people are on the road to recovery, they will understand this is a progressive service and they can keep on going.

Now, once they have obtained the 52 eClasses, of course they have them for life so they can keep going back and referring to them without requiring any further payments. What we cover:

The causes and development of Parkinson's.

How the disorder affects our body, our cells and cell interaction

All the self-help strategies we talk about

Food: what helps us; what harms us

Remedies and Therapies

Managing medication

Relating to health care practitioners

Gaining support from family and friends

Exercise

And all those aspects of the journey

There is quite a bit of free content on the website. Anyone interested can go and get a good look – a bit of a taste – of what we offer before they sign up.

I want to emphasize that health is an individual responsibility. My way is not the only way to recover from Parkinson's or to be well. It happens to be one way that has been proven because several people have recovered and many are becoming well.

It is a very individual choice. I think every individual has to ask a lot of questions, do a lot of research. Yes, it is good to be skeptical, but in the end choose what resonates and feels right and dedicate yourself to the process of becoming well, and expressing innate joyfulness and beauty.

Do you have any information regarding the supplement NADH that is supposed to improve cognitive abilities? Does it interfere with Azilect (or Rasagiline)?

I looked at NADH some years ago because it certainly has good press. I could not find any really positive support with regard to treating Parkinson's Disease.

While there are a number of supplements on the market that theoretically should help, when it comes down to practice, they do not seem to. When we trialed NADH with a number of my clients over a six month period we found no advantage in taking it. So, that is number one.

Azilect is not a particularly nice drug to be taking anyway. It is an MAO-B inhibitor (we think). Nobody is actually sure. The warning I have here is "the precise mechanisms of action of Azilect (Rasagiline) are unknown". One mechanism is believed to be related to its MAOB inhibitory activity. We do not know how it works.

In practice I have found that MAOB inhibitors (if Rasagiline is one) are not particularly useful. The other thing we need to look at is adverse effects and whether they overwhelm or offset any positive effects we might see.

There is a warning with Azilect that treatment with any dose may be associated with a hypertensive crisis if a patient ingests Tyramine with foods, beverages or dietary supplements or amines. Tyramine is present in many, many foods and we do not always know we are ingesting them.

There is a potential for dying from taking Rasagiline. Tyramine foods include:

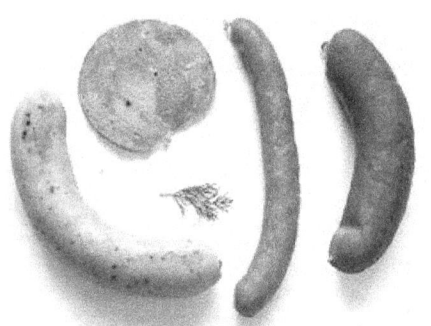

- Dried aged and fermented meats

- Fish

- Sausages

- Salamis

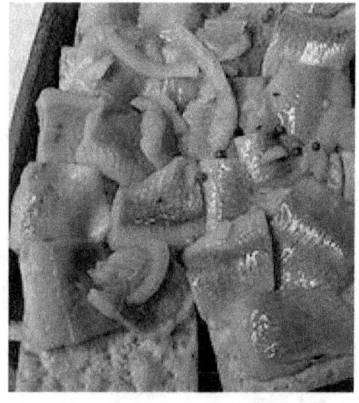

- Herring

- Any food that is slightly spoiled

- Broad beans

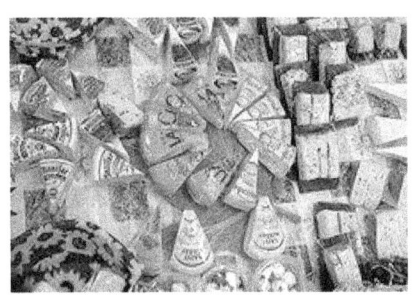

Aged cheeses

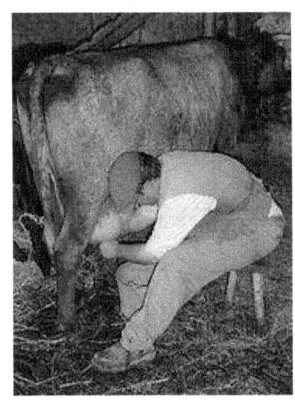

Dairy products

Tapped beers and beers that have not been   pasteurized

Concentrated juice extracts and overripe fruit

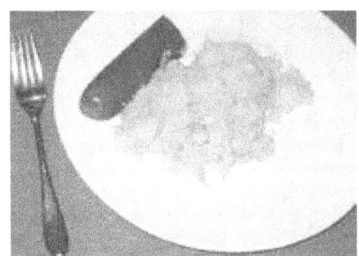

Sauerkraut

Soy bean products

There are a lot of foods that we need to avoid if we are taking Rasagiline anyway.

There are a number of adverse effects including nausea, headache, dizziness, depression, falling, conjunctivitis, fever, neuritis, rhinitis, arthritis, malaise, general feeling of illness, neck pain, vertigo, etc. It is not a particularly nice drug. It does not do a lot of good. Whether NADH is going *to react to it or not I am not sure but, in my opinion, neither of them is particularly useful.*

I was diagnosed with Parkinson's three and a half years ago. Currently I have rigidity with muscle spasms and uncomfortable sensations. My legs are heavy and my body drags while walking. My arms do not swing as they once did. Movement in my neck is restricted and painful. Throughout the day I feel rigidity, spasms and body sensations which are very disturbing.

I have subscribed to Dr. Coleman's 12 Step Recovery Program and now regularly take Aquas. I drink 8-10 glasses of water, do Bowen therapy and observe all possible dietary restrictions. But, still my neurological situation is aggregating.

> ### How can I reduce or manage my rigidity, spasms and burning sensations? Please advise me.

We need to have a look at the timing and some other supplements. We know that Parkinson's or the symptoms of Parkinson's begin in early childhood. Without knowing how old the person is who asked this question, we can conjecture it has taken at least 50-60 years for this condition to develop. Therefore, it will take some time for this condition to reverse. That is number one.

You have taken some sensible steps in beginning the journey with the Aquas and changing your diet. We need to be assiduous with that.

It is not usual that we get an aggravation of symptoms. However, it is common that in the first two months or so of going on the 12 Step Recovery Program we do not actually stop development of what is already going on.

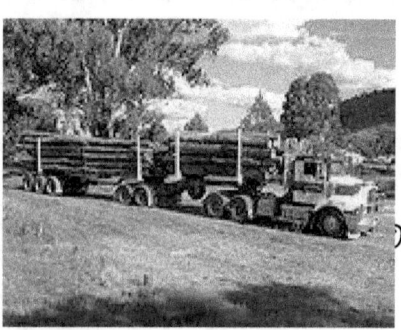

It is like stopping a large truck. When we put the brakes on it is still going to take 1,200

yards for the truck to actually pull up. So, you have started by putting the brakes on but it is taking a while for the symptoms to slow down and plateau.

However, there are some strategies we can look at. One is magnesium[1]. Magnesium is a <u>muscle relaxant</u> and also a nerve relaxant. It is used for brain cell function. I have found that one of the best ways to take magnesium as a supplement is in powder form.

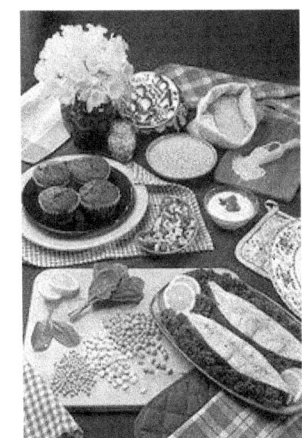

I would suggest that (although I do not know your level of sensitivity) if you get some powdered magnesium and start with about a half level teaspoon in a glass of water morning and evening. This can also be part of your water intake.

Slowly increase that dosage of magnesium until you may reach around a teaspoon morning and evening. The level that you choose will depend on what sort of muscle response you get and also what sort of bowel response you get. Magnesium in powered form is very useful if there is any bowel restriction at all.

If that is not sufficient to alleviate the symptoms to some degree then we need to look at how well your Bowen therapist is treating you – not that I am criticizing in any way – but sometimes we can

undertake other strategies as a Bowen therapist to relieve stiffness rigidity and that heavy feeling.

[1] **The picture to the right depicts food sources of magnesium**

33

You could ask your Bowen therapist to contact me for discussion about a process called <u>Tui Na</u> (around the feet) which is a very ancient Chinese therapy that combines very well with Bowen therapy to help alleviate neuro symptoms.

We also need to look at your exercise regime also – I do not think you mentioned this in your question. If you are walking, great, but specific exercises that are in some <u>yoga</u> modalities or in <u>Pilates</u> can also be very beneficial in alleviating the symptoms of spasm and stiffness and heaviness. So, there are a whole lot of strategies we can look at. If you have ongoing challenges I would be happy to hear from you.

How many people have undertaken the same plan and what results have they gotten?

Over the last 10 years I have treated something in excess of 2000 people with Parkinsons, a large percentage of them are from Australia but many are overseas. The level of success has depended primarily on the level of dedication that is brought to the process.

Of those who are really dedicated four have completely recovered. That is, they no longer have any Parkinson's symptoms at all. Their general health has improved significantly and they no longer use any Parkinson's medications.

- *A very significant number have improved their symptoms.*

- *Their symptoms have reduced.*

- *They are more functional.*

- *They are more comfortable.*

- *They have reduced their levels of medication.*

A number have stayed about the same. Some have gone on and continued to degenerate.

The interesting thing is that, when I first interview people and/or get their questionnaires, I ask for their feelings about what they want to achieve and what their goals are. Many people say to me,

> *"If I do not get any worse, I will be happy."*

And so, that is what they get. They don't get any worse but they also do not get any better because their goal is fixed on staying the same.

Other people will say to me,

> *"I want to be like I was before I got Parkinsons."*

They focus on that and that is what they get. The people who made the goal of making each day better and enjoying life to the full every moment, and who embraced the knowledge that they can improve their health, have gone on to get well

I saw a woman - one of my clients – Wednesday morning Melbourne time. She was diagnosed with Parkinson's 17 years ago. She came to see me about 9 years ago.

- *She has plodded on.*

- *She has maintained her spirit of determination.*

- *Her family has been supportive.*

- *She has gone on working with the Aquas and Bowen and supplements and we have looked at diet and her mindset.*

This is also a lady who struggles with English, so there has been some social isolation or communication difficulties here. Her condition in the last 12 months has improved by over 50%. So, she has attained a breakthrough. She has been on a plateau for years and now -

- *She has turned it around.*

- *She is actually getting better.*

- *She is walking better.*

- *She is standing better.*

- *She has reduced her medication.*

- *She has less anxiety*

- *She has less depression.*

- *She is sleeping better*

This is the sort of dedication it takes. We need to be focused on the fact that

- *we can get well*

- *We can improve our health.*

- *It is our responsibility*

And it is a long-term project.

At what point of noticing Parkinsonian symptoms says you have Parkinson's disease?

> *This is a very interesting question, because many symptoms we associate with PD are also associated with other so called diseases. I would like to make the point here that I do not believe in separate diseases. In my view, and in the view of many scientists in the world*

now, there is a degenerative process in our body that may manifest as a whole variety of symptoms that could be diagnosed as:

- *Cardiovascular disease or*

- *Diabetes or*

- *Cancer or*

- *Multiple Sclerosis or*

- *Motor Neurone Disease (ALS) or*

- *Lupus or*

- *Parkinson's Disease.*

There are symptoms that are common to many of those. The most common symptoms for PD are tremor of a particular kind - tremor at rest with pill rolling action - that affects about 60% or so of people diagnosed with Parkinson's. There is:

- *Slowing of movement,*

- *Paucity of movement*

- *Mask like expression*

- *Often a dragging of one leg*

- *One arm stops swinging appropriately*

- *There is a criterion of unilateral onset, that is, the onset of symptoms on one side and slow onset.*

In the end there is no test or point when we can say definitely we have Parkinson's disease. What we can say is you have a set of symptoms that seem to be Parkinson's.

We have done an MRI scan.

We have undertaken coordination and functional testing.

We have done the questionnaire.

We have eliminated the possibility of <u>Wilson's Disease</u> of toxicity – such as lead or manganese or cadmium.

We have eliminated the possibility of head stroke or head injury.

We have determined you are not taking any drugs that cause the symptoms.

So, we have to assume that you have Parkinson's. That is as good as it gets as far as diagnosis is concerned.

When should we start taking medication?

I believe there is only one class of drugs that is useful for treating Parkinson's and that is the <u>Levodopa</u> drugs. They are really very useful. They have generally controllable adverse effects.

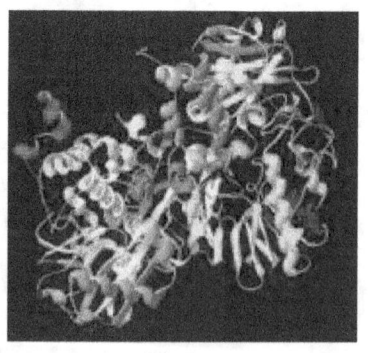

The COMT inhibitors, the <u>MAO inhibitors</u>, the <u>dopamine</u> all have pretty uncontrollable adverse effects. The <u>Levodopa</u> drugs have been proven to be useful functionally. The packaged inhibiter, like Carbidopa with Sinemet, assists in delivering the Levodopa to the brain optimally.

Interview with John Coleman, ND

I believe we should only take medication if our lack of function is such that it has become too uncomfortable or dangerous to carry out our daily tasks. If we are working for income for instance, it may be that our current symptoms inhibit our activity to a degree that we can't give good value for the money we are earning, and this is stressful for us. Levodopa is very useful in this case.

Or, Levodopa is very useful if we are moving around the house and we fall or we can't manage getting around the furniture or work in the kitchen.

However, I believe it needs to be used at a low dose. I believe we can start at 50 ml twice to three times a day This is assuming that we are also taking responsibility for our own health, making sure that our diet is great and our exercise is great and you are drinking water, etc.

If the 50 ml three times a day is not sufficient (and we need to try that for 6-8 weeks) then we can slowly increase it to say 100 ml. three times a day. I see clients who have managed with that level of medication for 5-6 years and are now starting to turn their symptoms around and come back to a much healthier state.

I may have given the impression during these questions or answers that recovery essentially takes 6-10 years. That is not necessary so. Of the people who have fully recovered, one took 2 and a half years and one took over 6 years. My recovery was over a period of about three and a half years. So, there is a wide range of times.

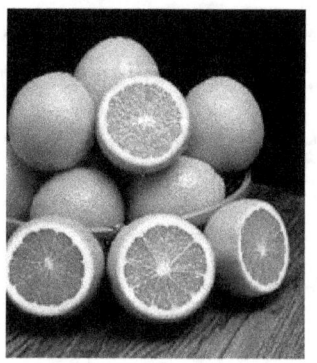

And needless to say, much depends on the level of dedication. The Levodopa during these times can be useful. If we are taking it we need to be taking good quantities of <u>Vitamin c</u> (4000 to 6000 milligrams daily) and <u>folic acid</u> (at least 500 microgram daily) to mop up the <u>homocysteine</u> we produce in our brain as a result of using Levodopa medication.

Could you discuss the approaches using the <u>Emotional Freedom Technique</u> for my Parkinson's condition and your opinion of the value of the technique?

This is a great question. <u>Emotional Freedom Technique</u> is a very simple and powerful technique for assisting us to turn negative emotions to a positive view. The technique was developed from <u>force field therapy</u> which is a much more complex process. Emotional Freedom Technique is very powerful and has been used around the world for years. It is one of a whole gamut of strategies we can use to develop a positive emotional status in our bodies.

The development of Parkinson's revolves around the non-resolution of trauma or high stress early in life. What that tends to do is get locked into our bodies so that our <u>response</u> to other situations is on the basis of fight, flight or freeze.

When we are dealing with the physical aspects of Parkinson's we also need to look at its emotional and spiritual aspects. That usually means we need to get fright out of our bodies so that our bodies can begin to produce _neurotransmitters_ appropriately and reduce the production of _stress_. That requires us to undertake strategies like:

- _Meditation_

- _Relaxation_

- _Walking_

- _Sitting_

- _Dreaming_

- _Singing_

- _Sleeping_

- _Listening to music_

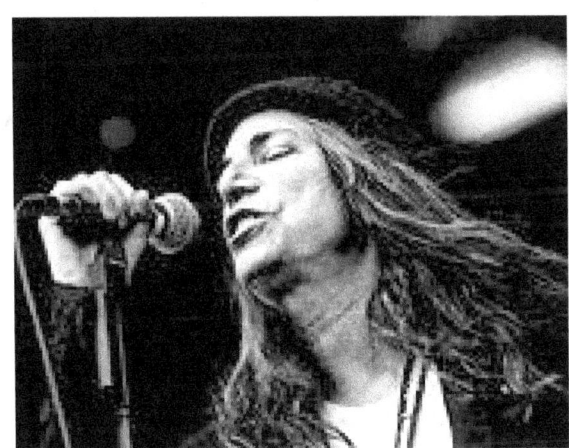

One of the strategies we can use is Emotional Freedom Technique (EFT). It has been a very powerful impact on a number of my clients. I have used it myself. My wife Nichol[2] has used it for a number of situations.

It is one of those strategies that can be used on a regular basis if we need to or just as and when we need. For instance, we can use EFT when we face a stressful situation or when we have a challenge in our minds as when one of those negative ideas goes

- _around and_
  - _around and_
- _around and_
  - _around._

---

[2] _Nichol stands next to John Coleman on the picture shown on the first page of this interview._

We can use EFT to break that cycle to develop a positive affirmation. There is a lot about EFT on the internet and it is really worth looking at and using from time to time or on a regular basis.

I take Mirapex three times a day; also Carbidopa/levodopa three times a day. Which should be taken first and when? How critical is the timing of taking medication?

The traditional view of dosing medication is that you need to take a very strict dose at exactly the same time each day, three times a day. There are usually very clear directions on the drugs as to whether there is going to be any interaction.

In practice over the last 10 years, I find that there is in fact a great deal of flexibility about medication dosage and timing. We can judge the timing and the amount of medication we take according to how we are feeling on any particular day - physically emotionally and spiritually - and what there is ahead for us that day.

For instance, clients I see quite regularly may be on a standard dose of 100 ml of Levodopa three times a day. However, the daily function varies significantly. So, if they are having a quiet day and they might be preparing a couple of meals they will 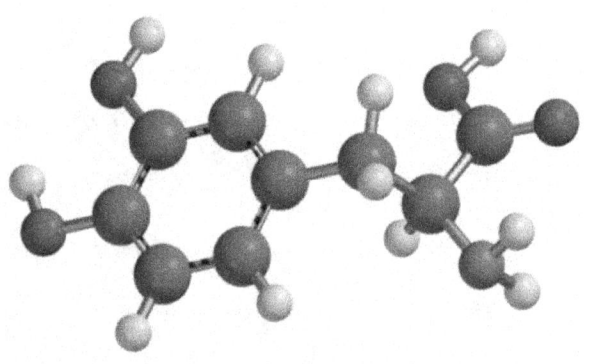 *generally take their first dose of medication around 8 o'clock or so in the morning. Then they may take 50 ml instead of 100 ml sometime after lunch. That might be all they need.*

Interview with John Coleman, ND

On the other hand, some of my clients have part time work. On the days they go to work they get up early.

- *They take the first 100 ml of Levodopa at 6:30 or 7:00.*

- *They get ready for work.*

- *They go to work.*

- *At 12:00 or 12:30 they take 100 ml of Levodopa.*

When they get home from work at 5:30 or 6:00 o'clock then they decide:.

- *Do they need another dose?*

- *Do they need 50 ml?*

- *Do they need 100 ml?*

That depends on how well they are functioning, whether the day has been stressful or pretty easy and whether the dose allows them to do their duties.

There are occasions - rare occasions – where they may have worked all day and have to go out at night. They will take an extra 50 ml to get them through. Occasionally they take none.

To me, this is a sensible use of medication. The days when they take less it gives their bodies a chance to produce more dopamine and more Serotonin

Please remember this. Don't be locked into the myth that the symptoms of Parkinson's disease means we only have a deficiency of Dopamine. Studies here and around the world have indicated that there are roughly 43 neurotransmitters deficient when we produce symptoms of Parkinsons.

These include _Anandamide_ _Serotonin_, _Dopamine_, _Glutamine_ and _Melatonin_ as well as a whole bunch of other neurotransmitters[3].

When we reduce the level of medication in our bodies any day our body is more active in producing _neurotransmitters_ endogenously or within the body. But on the days when we need some extra support it is ok to take that extra medication because we are using it according to our need for function.

In theory you need to take it strictly according to prescribed dose and prescribed time. In practice it can be variable in both cases.

How do I handle the negativity (Doomsday) when keeping my appointment with the neurologist?

This is a challenge that we all face, and there are a couple of strategies that I can suggest and I think you could look at. I am not saying every one of these needs to be your strategy.

Number One: How important is it to see your neurologist? What do you want from your neurologist?

- _Do you want a prescription for drugs? Get it from your general practitioner._

- _Do you want an assessment or your condition? Be prepared then for a negative report._

- _Do you want to develop a rapport and companionship? Forget it. It is not going to happen._

Let's say that you feel you feel need to make annual or bi annual visits to your neurologist for particular reasons. The number one strategy is to

---

[3] _The picture on page 20 depicts neurons in human hippocampal tissue._

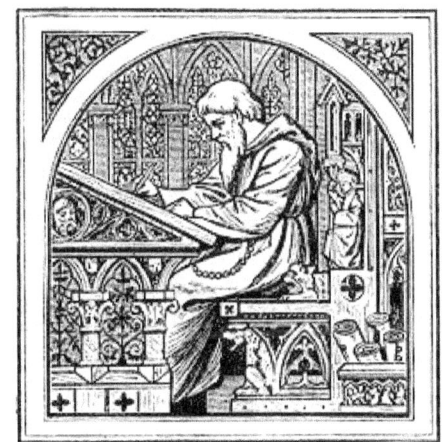

prepare yourself in writing. That is, if you have questions to ask, write those questions down and make a copy so that you have a copy and there is a copy to hand to your neurologist. If you feel that you have stabilized or you have made some improvements, write that down and hand a copy of that report to your neurologist too.

When he or she starts on the –

"Well, um … we need to increase your medication."

Then, you say:

"No. I want you to look at areas in my life that have actually improved. I would like you to focus on those."

As far as the doomsday predictions, this is what neurologists know. This is what they are taught. They have 12 years of medical school. Teaching them that illness is the most important thing in life and they have the unique power to treat illness and if they cannot treat illness nobody else can.

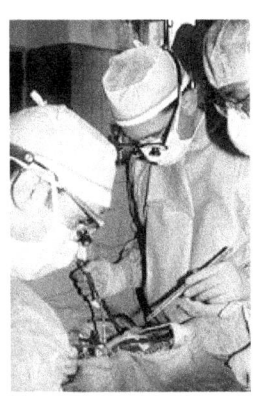

"Nobody can do anything for themselves."

Is what they learn. Then, after the 12 years of medical school and internship, they are exposed to a whole bunch of learning about neurology. They learn about illness. That is all they learn about; illness and controlling illness.

Interview with John Coleman, ND

They are unfortunate people because they learn nothing about wellness, about positiveness or about self-responsibility. It is not in their training. So, we can feel sorry for them.

I say ignore predictions because we know their predictions are wrong. We know that for any doctors or, for that matter, any naturopath, prognosis is a best guess. When a doctor says to somebody – you have cancer – you will be dead in six months. That is a best guess. What we do is take that on as gospel truth and we die in six months to prove them right, but we don't have to.

When doctors say to us – you have Parkinson's disease, you will get worse, you will need Apomorphine subcutaneously., you will need a wheel chair, you will need full time care - these are all best guesses. We do not have to prove it is true. We do not have a responsibility to prove that the doctor is right.

Our responsibility is to us. I think we need to write this down.

> "I am the most important person in my life. I create my own prognosis."

So we need to build ourselves up. I think is also important, whenever going to a neurologist, to take a buddy with us, whether that is:

- a spouse or

- a partner or

- a close friend or

- a child or

- *a sibling*

1. *Someone who is attached to you.*

2. *Someone who is feeling positive about your taking control of your life and is very encouraging about that.*

3. *Someone who will be your ears.*

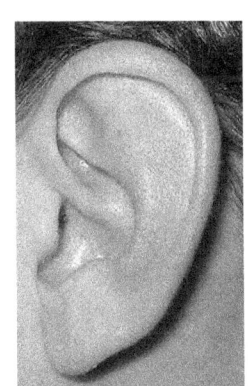

They can sit back and listen and focus on what you are saying and what the neurologist is saying. Often we hear the bad stuff and that overwhelms us. We don't hear some of the good stuff.

Sometimes perhaps the neurologist is saying strongly:

> *"Look you are going to get worse and you need to increase medication."*

They might be saying quietly,

> *"I do not understand why you haven't got worse."*

That has happened to some of my clients. The emphasis is still on what they know – that is, that people get worse. A buddy with you can help hear those puzzled statements from the neurologist or if the neurologist is a bully – some are – not many – then you have someone there to support you and encourage you to communicate your concerns.

Here In Australia, there are few neurologists who are quite positive in outlook. I know of four here in Melbourne. There is another further up in the gold coast and one in Sydney. While they are not knowledgeable about complementary medicine, they are encouraging to their patients and say:

- *Yes, you can do things for yourself.*

- *Yes, it is good to meditate.*

- *Yes, it is good to see a naturopath.*

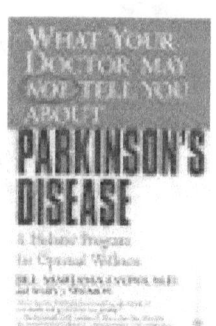

I am hopeful that there is one or more in your area. I know there is neurologist in Florida, Jill Marjama-Lyons[4], who wrote a book (with Mary Shomon) called What Your Doctor May Not Tell You About Parkinson's. She is quite amenable to things like meditation and supplements.

You may find it better to look around for a neurologist who is a bit more supportive even if not directly knowledgeable about complementary medicine.

In closing, when you go to a neurologist, expect they will speak from their very limited knowledge base. Take from them what you want and forget their prognosis. If they push you to increase medication, make up your own mind. It may not be necessary.

In Your 12 Step Recovery Program, are some steps more important than others?

Yes, there are. Let's have a look at the key steps.

Step 1: Understanding How Parkinson's Disease Develops

I believe is really important, the more we know about why our body is behaving in a particular way – the greater the power we have to turn that around. If we truly understand how and why we develop

---

[4] *Department of Physical Therapy, Box 100154, University of Florida, Gainesville, FL 32610-0154, USA*

Parkinson's disease, we can realize we have an enormous amount of power to change this.

- *It is not something we catch.*

- *It is not something mysterious.*

- *It is not beyond our understanding.*

- *It is a simply, well understand process of suppressing the fight-flight response.*

Step 2 - Loving Ourselves.

This is probably the most important step of all because everything else can revolve around that. If we truly love ourselves:

- *We will eat food that is good for us.*

- *We will avoid destructive behavior.*

- *We will have far more positive thought processes and far less negative ones and can change the negative ones*

- *We will undertake exercise that enhances our well being.*

- *We will visit practitioners who treat us respectfully and lovingly and support us in our journey.*

So loving ourselves: In the 12 Step Recovery Program I give ways that we can do this – loving ourselves really is the basis of turning our health around.

Interview with John Coleman, ND

Step 5 – Laughter[5]

I have a concept – the3L's – Love, Laughter and Meditation. I hope everyone is laughing because meditation does not start with the letter L. It is something I concocted.

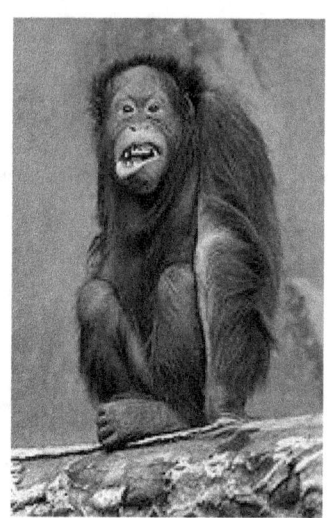

Laughter is the second string of this real basis of us turning our health around. When we laugh or pretend to laugh we produce Anandamide, Dopamine and Serotonin and we reduce the production of stress hormones. Step 5 is also a really important one.

Step 7 – Meditating.

Meditation is really simple. It is a practice that is as old as man.

- *We would meditate in our cave or place of sleep*

- *We would drink in the sun and we would consider that strengthening*

- *We would worship whatever we would worship.*

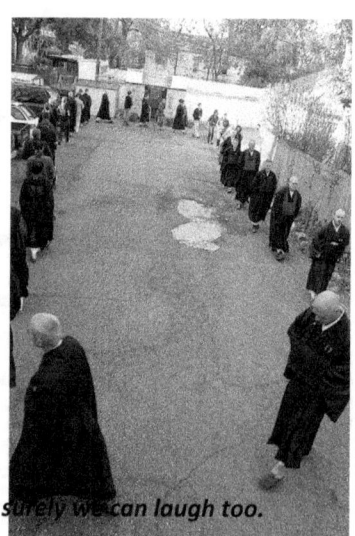

These are all forms of mediation. We all mediate during our lives when we see things of great beauty or great peace.

---

[5] **Picture shows an Orangutan laughing. If a monkey can laugh, surely we can laugh too.**

So those four steps: step 2, step 5 and step 7 are the bases. Step 1 is very, very important.

Step 6 – Diet

This is really absolutely critical. If we truly love ourselves as I said, we will eat the food that is good for us. Sometimes we get confusing messages about that. So, in step 6 – and I think there are actually 3 e-classes I have written on that - diet provides the body with fuel that supports our loving ourselves.

Does your 12 Step Recovery Program interfere or complement electric Deep Brain Stimulation (DBS)?

This opens a real can of worms for you. DBS is being used more and more. There is I think something like 20,000 people who have undertaken this process. In general I would say it has been a dismal failure.

However, if someone has had that surgery and is struggling with their health – as most are – then the 12 Step Recovery Program or the program I promote can assist in improving their health. I have found with those people who have come to me following DBS that it is much more difficult to become fully well because there is very significant damage to the brain by the surgery itself. I know that, theoretically, there are just two very thin wires being inserted very deep into the brain in two very specific areas. Those wires happen to kill several million

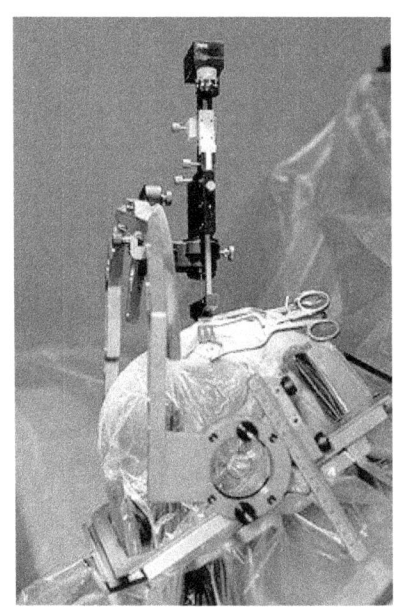

51

cells on the way in. We also have electrical discharge into the brain. This seems to disrupt some function.

What I have seen, as a result, is that some people gain immediate improvement and are really happy about it. And over the next 15 months to 3 years they start to deteriorate. They move back onto drugs.

There is a neurologist by the name of David Heydrick who has DBS and has managed, through exercise, diet and really positive thinking, to move away from his medication. Mind you he still has very serious symptoms of Parkinsons.

I have seen his DVD. People who are considering DBS need to consider it again and again, and I would certainly not undertake it unless and until you have met several people who have had DBS at least 5 years ago at least.

I recently had an interview with Richard Moir[6]. Richard is an Australian actor who developed Parkinson's disease many, many years ago. He came to see me several times but could not develop the dedication and determination to actually get well. He was on high medication, Apomorphine subcutaneously. He was a young man in his forties.

He decided to undergo DBS and made a movie about it called The Bridge at Midnight Trembles. That is available as a DVD[7]. It is worth looking at. It shows his condition before and following DBS.

---

[6] **Richard Moir** *(born 1950) is a Queensland-born Australian actor. In 1990, Moir was diagnosed with Parkinson's Disease, the degenerative effects of which gradually brought his acting career to a premature end. Moir later underwent deep brain stimulation therapy, a process covered by the 2006 documentary The Bridge At Midnight Trembles*

[7] **Find reviews at** http://www.peterleiss.com/html/films_reviews2.html

Interview with John Coleman, ND

His body function certainly does improve to some degree following DBS. He had a nightmare ride in having surgery, infection, adjusting the electrical discharge to reach the stage of semi functionality with drug support.

Following that he has actually had 6 more <u>DBS</u> surgeries and has had 7 in total. He is an absolute mess. He is making another movie called The Wind Howls Like a Hammer! about his experiences. These are going to be good movies to watch if you are considering having <u>DBS.</u>

The movies I have seen from the medical profession show the instant benefits. Maybe 50 % of the people experience instant benefits and some short term. In the long term however I have yet to see success.

That makes sense to me because what we have done is put a bandage on the electrical discharge in the brain that is deteriorating. The process of having many MRI's, local anesthetics, the trauma of having your skull cut open, etc., also exacerbates the symptoms of Parkinson's. So, we try the opposite of something that can be helpful.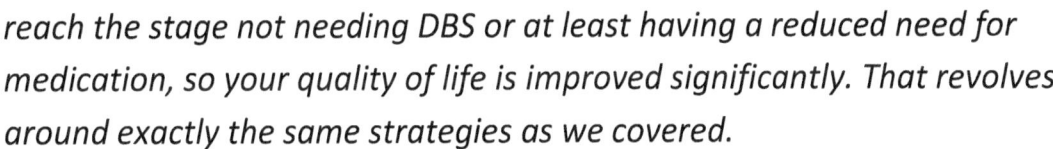

All of that being said is – if you have already had DBS, you can improve your health and you can possibly reach the stage not needing DBS or at least having a reduced need for medication, so your quality of life is improved significantly. That revolves around exactly the same strategies as we covered.

> **Given that you worked in a copper mine at age 16 suggests metal poisoning caused your Parkinson's. A chemist says, once rid of the metal, your body recovered. Most don't have such a traceable cause. Your method healed you, yet may not transfer to others?**

We know that heavy metals can be an exacerbating factor in developing of Parkinson's disease and Parkinson's symptoms. It is true that I worked in a copper mine. However my contact with cooper was minimal. I worked first worked as a clerk and then as a timekeeper.

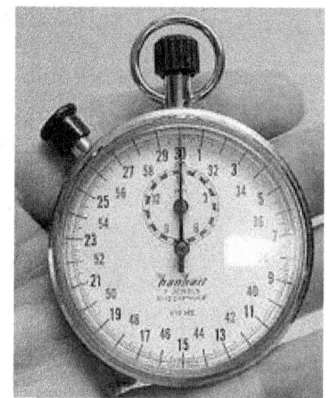

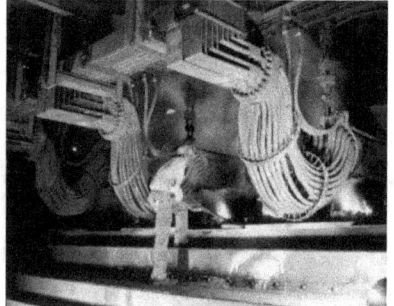

I had significant contact with the crude ore but not with copper per se which was down in the smelter. There were also other pollutants - the smelter pollutants. This was certainly a factor that we looked at.

We looked for Wilson's Disease of course that is an ingestion and collection of copper[8]. We looked at heavy metals. In fact, we could not find heavy metals. We looked for lead because I grew up in the era of leaded pipes. My Dad was a builder. Often there was a lot of paint around but we could not find lead toxicity either.

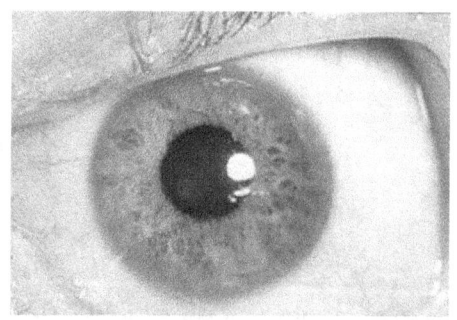

---

[8] *Picture of the eye shows a Kayser-Fleischer ring in a patient with symptoms suggestive of Wilson's disease*

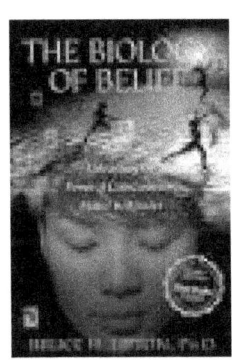

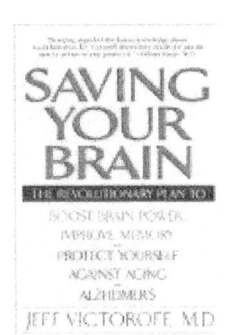

More telling than that is that we know what causes Parkinson's. This is now unequivocal. When we read studies by Jeff Victoroff, Bruce McEwen, Gabor Mate and Bruce Lipton among others, we know that, like all degenerative disorders, Parkinson's begins in early childhood with a suppression of the fight-flight response. This might occur as a result of many, many different types of circumstances.

When we are already in this state of suppressed fight-flight response, other toxins can have a greater impact on us. They may include copper garden sprays such as Diazinon[9] and Roundup, it may include things like lead or cadmium or dry cleaning fluids[10] or paint or any number of other chemicals that are around. Even petroleum and diesel (gas in your world) may create and exacerbate symptoms.

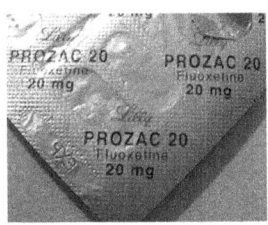

Certain drugs can do that also. Amiodarone is one – a drug

---

[9] *Diazinon kills insects by inhibiting acetylcholinesterase, an enzyme necessary for proper nervous system function. Diazinon has a low persistence in soil. The half-life is 2 to 6 weeks.[1] The symptoms associated with diazinon poisoning in humans include weakness, headaches, tightness in the chest, blurred vision, nonreactive pinpoint pupils, excessive salivation, sweating, nausea, vomiting, diarrhea, abdominal cramps, and slurred speech.*

[10] **Like many chlorinated hydrocarbons, tetrachloroethene (or dry cleaning fluid) is a central nervous system depressant, and inhaling its vapors (particularly in closed, poorly ventilated areas) can cause dizziness, headache, sleepiness, confusion, nausea, difficulty in speaking and walking, unconsciousness, and death.**

given for _arrhythmias_ is known to produce Parkinsonian symptoms as do the _Lipitrophic_ drugs[11]. The Lipitor _cholesterol drugs_ they are very, very toxic drugs and can cause and exacerbate Parkinson's symptoms as can _anti-depressants_.

The fact is our brain is already set up to be vulnerable. This is where we need to look at how our Parkinson's starts. Yes, we need to be aware that toxic chemicals and metals are going to have an influence on our life. You may need to move away from an area or clean our body out gently. Detoxes must always be gentle.

We need to look at how our Parkinson's began. It always comes up as a suppression of the _fight flight_ response and that is where we start our work.

> **Over the last few days there have been results of studies suggesting that there can be benefits of early medication rather than delaying medication. Comments?**

I find that very difficult to accept. I have not seen the studies, However we know that the focus of medication – whether it be _Levodopa_ medication, _dopamine_, _MAO-B inhibitors_, COMT inhibitors and _Anti-cholinergic_ drugs - is on improving the quantity of available _dopamine_ in the brain.

Two things here are happening. When we do that we reduce or suppress the ability of our body to produce endogenous dopamine. We ignore the deficiency of other _neurotransmitters_ involved as in Anandamide, _Serotonin_ and _Glutamine_

---

[11] Common _adverse drug reactions_ (≥1% of patients, or more than one out of every one hundred patients) associated with atorvastatin therapy include: _myalgia_, mild transient gastrointestinal symptoms (diarrhea, constipation, passing gas), elevated hepatic _transaminase_ concentrations, headache, insomnia, joint pain, and/or dizziness.[4]

Interview with John Coleman, ND

The earlier we introduce medications, the more likely it is that down the track we will have both adverse reactions and ineffective medication, and a rapidly exacerbating disorder.

We have an increasing ratio of young onset Parkinson's being diagnosed these days. I believe this is definitely as a result of a very toxic society.

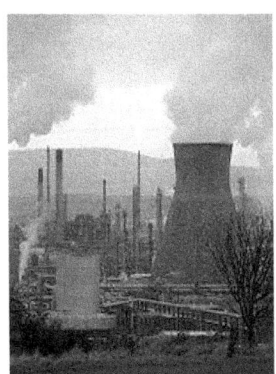

- *Very poor food.*

- *Toxic food with lots of petrochemicals with coloring and flavorings.*

- *The huge influx of artificial sweeteners which are highly neuro toxic.*

- *The influx of petroleum traffic and industrial pollution,*

- *Fluoride in water*

All play a role in the development of degenerative disorders. I would encourage us to look at not using medication unless we need it. As I say, where function is difficult and at all dangerous, then Levodopa medication is the best.

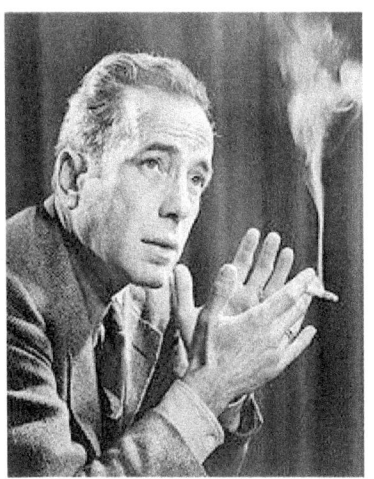

I also need to warn is against the study that looks at the effect of smoking on the symptoms of Parkinson's. There are a number of studies that say smoking cigarettes delays the onset if Parkinson's. That is a load of rubbish. A study will show this, but it was constructed in such a way that it had to show that.

In fact, what we know happens is that smoking

cigarettes (that is, ingesting nicotine) disguises the onset of Parkinsons. It fools our body into believing that it has more dopamine, Serotonin and Glutamine than it actually has because nicotine occupies those receptors.

It is similar to ingesting cannabis or smoking marijuana. Cannabis occupies receptors intended for Anandamide. Anandamide is the neurotransmitter that makes us feel fabulous and makes every cell in our body work better.

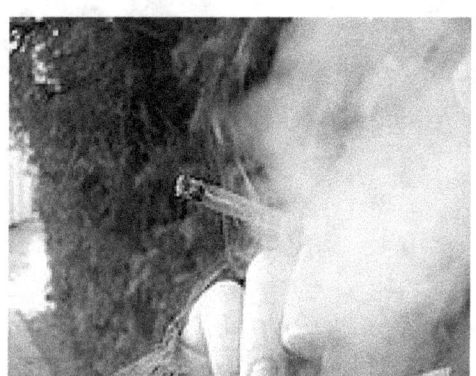

There is a lot of information on Anandamide on the internet that is worth looking at. Anandamide was discovered when people were looking for the mechanism of cannabis and how that worked in the body.

When we smoke cannabis it makes us feel fabulous I am told. I have never used it. It is supposed to give us the feeling of euphoria, but it discourages the production of Anandamide and incidentally Dopamine and Serotonin in the body. Early ingestion of Parkinson's medication - even dopamine and things like Selegiline – are likely to exacerbate the disorder down the track in 10 or 15 years. I do disagree with that study and warn against that and say – look for more information.

How long did it take you see substantial symptom relief? How long did it take to become symptom free?

I didn't see substantial symptom relief for a long time. What I saw were tiny improvements. I collapsed in August in 1995. The only reason I did not take medication was that I was treated dreadfully by medical practitioners, a couple of neurologists.

Interview with John Coleman, ND

I had two surgeons who worked with me, a neurosurgeon and another plastic surgeon who knew me and diagnosed Parkinson's and said to me

"Do not take medications unless you absolutely have to."

I battled on with a

- *Homeopath*

- *Counselor*

- *Craniosacral therapist*

By early 1996 after about 4-5 months I had seen some small improvements. I was almost coherent with my speech. I was speaking very slowly and pausing often, but I could get a sentence out. I could walk 100 meters or so providing I had support and 20 to 30 meters without support providing I focused. I could actually just do a day's work, so I had improved. I do not call that substantial improvement.

I did not see substantial improvement after that until late 1996 or early 1997 when I was well into this routine of diet, meditation and using homeopathics without necessarily understanding what I was doing. I seemed to be doing some of the right things.

In the middle of 1996 I had a huge setback. My back went into spasms I still do not know why. It has happened to other people. We are looking at that syndrome. I had enormous spasms for a couple of days.

59

© Parkinsons Reco

Interview with John Coleman, ND

That knocked me around for 2 or 3 months and put me back.

Then, towards the second half of 1997 I had another huge setback. I thought I was really worse than I was in 1995 and then battled out of that.

The total time from collapse in August in 1995 to symptom free in mid 1998 was three years. I thought I was well then but I realize I wasn't. I was just symptoms free.

I continued to work with my health and improved significantly. Today I have to say - 10 years since I became symptom free – I am much healthier than I was then. I am 10 years older, but

- *I walk further.*

- *I exercise more.*

- *I can work out.*

- *I feel better.*

My health has improved significantly in the 10 years. It was three years to become symptom free.

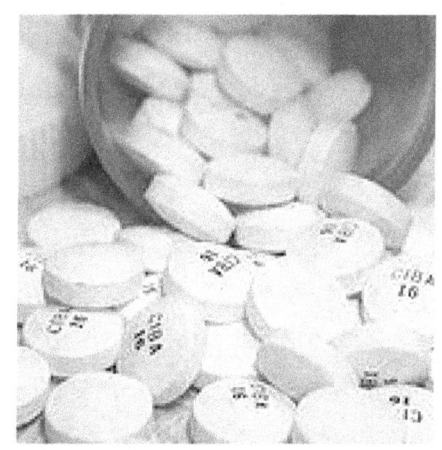

My first recovery client was a 79 year old man when he came to me from Queensland in Australia. He came to me at stage 4 and a half (there are 5 stages, with 5 being the worst). He collapsed on walking with a frame. He was on 1500 milligrams Levodopa a day plus 12-13 other drugs for various elements including Parkinson's, blood pressure, reflux etc.

He took about 6 and a half years before he became symptom free. He noticed improvements I think after 1 year 2 weeks and 11 days. He was able to leave his walking frame behind and go walking by himself without support for the first time in many years. That was a very substantial improvement.

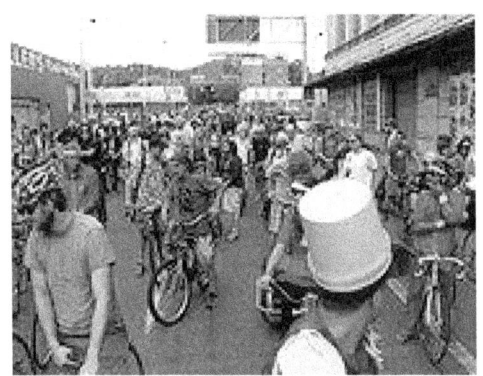

I think one of the secrets of getting well is to keep a journal

Keep a record of what is going on week by week and month by month so you can see very small improvements. I kept a diary and the very small improvements encouraged me to keep going so I was able to accumulate large improvements over a longer period of time.

Could you say a little about your *12 Step Recovery Program*?

I am really passionate about this. I know that you can get well.

1. *I got well.*

2. *Shelly got well.*

3. *Tom got well.*

4. *Elizabeth got well.*

5. *Harold got well.*

I am seeing improvements every week in my clients who have Parkinson's. I know this really works. Just with beginning the activities you will see some changes in your body.

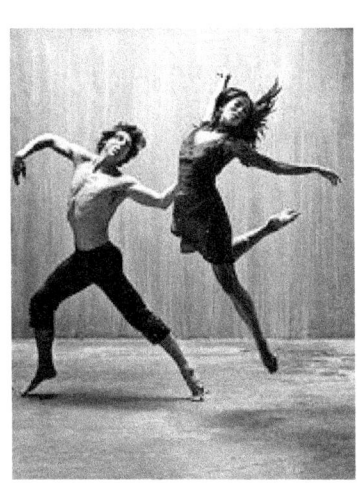

- *Nothing is impossible.*

- *We can get well.*

Interview with John Coleman, ND

- *People are recovering from Parkinsons.*

- *I encourage you to take control.*

- *Take responsibility.*

- *Know that you can get well.*

About Parkinsons Recovery

John Coleman was interviewed by Robert Rodgers, PhD, founder of **Parkinsons Recovery** which was established to provide information, support and resources to persons who currently experience symptoms of Parkinson's disease. This interview was originally published in the Pioneers of Recovery series published by Parkinsons Recovery.

Index

*12 Step Recovery Program, **32, 48, 49, 51, 61***

*abusive childhood, **6***

*adrenal glands, **18***

*adrenal stimulation, **15***

*adverse effects, **29, 31, 38***

*affirmations, **11, 16, 22***

*amino acids, **17***

*Amiodarone, **55***

*anandamide, **18***

*Anandamide, **44, 57, 58***

*Anandamides, **58***

*Anti-cholinergic, **56***

*Antidepressant therapy, **9***

*anti-depressants, **56***

*anxiety, **36***

*Anxiety, **14***

Interview with John Coleman, ND

Apomorphine, **46, 52**

Aquas, **12, 32, 35**

arrhythmias, **55**

artificial sweeteners, **57**

avocado, **12**

Azilect, **29, 30**

body drags while walking, **32**

bodywork, **9**

bowel dehydration, **17**

Bowen therapist, **33**

Bowen therapy, **32, 34**

Bowen Therapy, **13**

brain cell function, **33**

Bruce Lipton, **55**

Bruce McEwen, **55**

burning sensations, **32**

cadmium, **38, 55**

Cancer, **37**

cannabis, **57, 58**

Cardiovascular disease, **37**

Cdopa/ldopa, **42**

chamomilla, **15**

Chinese therapy, **33**

chiropractic, **9**

chiropractor, **5**

chiropractors, **8**

cholesterol drugs, **55**

cigarette smoker, **6**

cleaning fluids, **55**

coenzyme Q10, **8**

coffea, **15**

coffee, **13**

complementary medicine, **47, 48**

constipated, **7**

Constipation, **17**

copper mine, **53, 54**

counseling, **9, 22**

Counselor, **58**

counselors, **14**

Craniosacral therapist, **59**

cure, **10, 11**

dairy, **12**

David Heydrick, **52**

DBS, **51, 52, 53**

Deep Brain Stimulation, **51**

deep tissue massage, **9**

degenerative disorders, **55, 57**

depression, **9, 16, 17, 31, 36**

Diabetes, **37**

diagnosis, **19, 20, 21**

Diazinon, **55**

diet, **12, 17, 26, 32, 35, 39, 52, 59**

Diet, **51**

Dogwood, **15**

dopamine, **12, 18, 38, 43, 56, 57, 58**

Dopamine, **44, 50, 58**

dragging of one leg, **37**

Emotional Freedom Technique, **40, 41**

exercise, **11, 13, 15, 16, 17, 18, 26, 34, 39, 49, 52, 60**

fight, flight or freeze, **40**

fight-flight, **49, 55**

fight-flight response, **55**

fish, **12**

Fluoride, **57**

folic acid, **40**

force field therapy, **40**

freezing, **19**

fresh air, **15**

Gabor Mate, **21, 55**

gardening, **16**

gastrointestinal tract, **17**

Glutamine, **56, 57**

head stroke, **38**

headache, **13, 14**

heavy metals, **54**

herbalist, **17**

herbicides, **26**

Homeopath, **58**

homeopathic remedies, **9, 12, 13, 15**

homeopathics, **59**

homocysteine, **40**

Hops, **15**

hypothalamus, **12**

intermittent tremor, **5**

Jamaica, **15**

Jeff Victoroff, **21, 55**

Jill Marjama-Lyons, **48**

journal, **22, 61**

journals, **7, 22, 25**

kinesiologists, **14**

laughing, **12**

laughter, **13**

Laughter, **50**

lead, **38, 54, 55**

lead toxicity, **54**

Levodopa, **20, 38, 39, 40, 42, 43, 56, 57, 60**

lifestyle, **11, 24, 26**

Lupus, **37**

magnesium, **13, 15, 17, 33**

magnesium powders, **13**

manganese, **38**

MAO-B inhibitor, **29**

MAO-B inhibitors, **38, 56**

Mary Shomon, **48**

Mask like expression, **37**

mask-like face, **19**

Meditate, **13**

meditation, **11, 14, 15, 16, 22, 25, 48, 50, 59**

Meditation, **18, 41, 50**

melatonin, **15**

Melatonin, **44**

Melbourne, **35, 47**

mentoring program, **27**

Michael J. Fox, **20**

Mirapex, **42**

Mono Neuro disease, **37**

Motor Neurone disease, **37**

Interview with John Coleman, ND

MRI scan, **19, 38**

Muhammad Ali, **20**

Multiple Sclerosis, **37**

multiple system atrophy, **20**

muscle spasms, **32**

NADH, **29, 31**

naturopath, **10, 17**

naturopathy, **8**

neck is restricted and painful, **32**

neurologist, **44, 45, 46, 47, 48, 52**

neurology, **45**

neuroplasticity, 67, 68

neurosurgeon, **58**

neurotransmitters, **12, 16, 17, 41, 44, 56**

nicotine, **6, 57**

Norman Doidge, **21, 68**

Nulax, **17**

nutritional supplements, **9, 12, 14**

One arm stops swinging, **37**

osteopaths, **8**

pain, **7, 9, 13, 14, 15**

Passionflower, **15**

peristalsis movement, **17**

pesticides, **26**

petrochemicals, **57**

picnoginal, **8**

Pilates, **16, 18, 34**

pill rolling, **19, 37**

poor digestion, **17**

protein, **12**

Psychiatry, **9**

Queensland, **52, 60**

Rasagiline, **29, 30, 31**

Richard Moir, **52**

rigidity, **32, 33**

Selegiline, **58**

serotonin, **15, 18**

Serotonin, **43, 44, 50, 56, 58**

Sidney, **47**

Interview with John Coleman, ND

sleep, *14, 15, 16*

sleeping, *36*

slow movements, *19*

smelter pollutants, *54*

smoking, *57*

spasm, 34

spasms, *32, 59*

sports massage, *9*

stiffness, 34

Stop Parkin' and Start Livin', *12*

stress, *40, 41, 50*

stress hormones, *12, 18*

supplements, *8, 17, 29, 30, 32, 35, 48*

Sydney, *47*

symptom relief, *58*

symptoms, *5, 6, 9, 10, 11, 13, 14, 15, 16, 17, 18, 19, 20, 21, 22, 23, 24, 26, 32, 33, 34, 36, 37, 38, 39, 43, 52, 53, 54, 55, 57, 59*

Tai Chi, *16*

The Brain That Changes Itself: Stories of Personal Triumph from the frontiers of brain science, 67

The Bridge at Midnight Trembles, *52*

trauma, *40*, 53

Trauma, *14*

tremor, *6, 18, 19, 37*

Tremors, *18*

Tui Na, *33*

Tyramine, *30*

vegetables, *12*

visualization, *14*

visualizations, *16*

Vitamin c, *40*

Vitamin C, *8, 17*

Vitamin E, *8*

Walk, *13*

water, *13, 17*

What Your Doctor May Not Tell You About Parkinson's, *48*

wheat, *12*

*Wilson's Disease, **38, 54***

*yoga, **16, 17, 34***

Reference

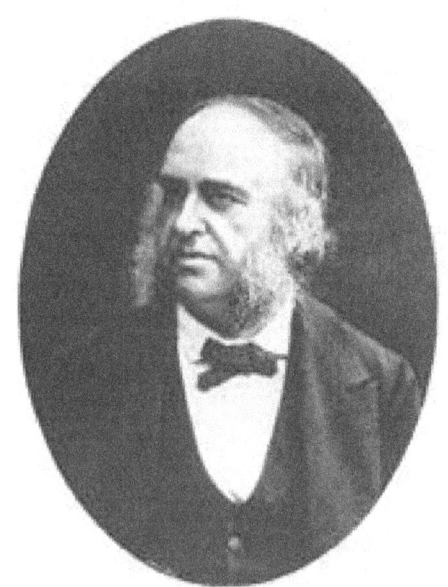

The Brain That Changes Itself: Stories of Personal Triumph from the frontiers of brain science *is a book on neuroplasticity by psychiatrist Norman Doidge M.D. It follows the lives of several medically injured patients and details just how the brain adapts to compensate for their disabilities.*